THE BREAST CANCER SURVIVOR'S DAILY QUOTE BOOK

Celebrating Life Every Day of the Year

by: Torran Bagamary and Michelle Iglesias

CCC Books

PO Box 1827

Westfield, MA 01086

by: Torran Bagamary and Michelle Iglesias

Copyright © 2008 CCC Books

Published in the U.S.A. by CCC Books

PO Box 1827, Westfield, MA 01086

(413) 205-8346

www.stillbeautifulstore.com

ISBN # 978-0-578-00846-2

In memory of Michael B. Lynn

and his three loving dogs,

Chewy, Chuck, and Chico

CONTENTS

INTRODUCTION

You are alive! Be thankful! Live life to the fullest! Don't just wait to celebrate the special occasions such as anniversaries, birthdays, Christmas, or any other holiday. If there is one thing that all survivors should have learned is that life is fragile, and that each day is special and worth rejoicing for. This is what this book offers you—a reason to celebrate every day you are alive. With 365 wise, warm, and witty words by philosophers, poets, novelists, comedians, and public figures, from Aristotle to Mark Twain, from Erma Bombeck to Oprah Winfrey, from Eleanor Roosevelt to Ralph Waldo Emerson, and many, many others, every page will inspire you to celebrate every day of the rest of your life. You fought the fight to survive, now celebrate more than ever that you are alive!

Michelle Iglesias

Wilbraham, Massachusetts

4 year survivor

JANUARY

JANUARY 1ST

The more you praise and celebrate your life,

the more there is in life to celebrate.

Oprah Winfrey

JANUARY 2ND

I like living. I have sometimes been wildly, despairingly,

acutely miserable, racked with sorrow, but through it all

I still know quite certainly

that just to be alive is a grand thing.

Agatha Christie

JANUARY 3RD

And in the end, it's not the years in your life that count.

It's the life in your years.

Abraham Lincoln

JANUARY 4th

Live life to the fullest.

Earnest Hemingway

JANUARY 5TH

Put yourself in a state of mind where you say to

yourself, "Here is an opportunity for you

to celebrate like never before, my own power, my own

ability to get myself to do

whatever is necessary."

Anthony Robbins

JANUARY 6TH

You will find as you look back upon your life

that the moments when you have really lived

are the moments when you have done things

in the spirit of love.

Henry Drummond

11

JANUARY 7TH

Nothing in life is to be feared.

It is only to be understood.

Marie Curie

JANUARY 8TH

Life has two rules:

number 1, Never quit!;

number 2, Always remember rule number 1.

Duke Ellington

JANUARY 9TH

I could not, at any age, be content to take my place

by the fireside and simply look on.

Life was meant to be lived.

Curiosity must be kept alive.

One must never, for whatever reason,

turn his back on life.

Eleanor Roosevelt

JANUARY 10TH

Our care should not be to have lived long

as to have lived enough.

Seneca

JANUARY 11TH

The greatest pleasure in life

is to do what people say you cannot do.

Walter Bagehot

JANUARY 12TH

Live as if you were to die tomorrow…

Learn as if you were to live forever.

Mahatma Gandhi

JANUARY 13TH

Life is best experienced with a sense of awe, wonder and

discovery. Go about life with a child's curiosity.

The universe is more spectacular than you can imagine.

Tom Gregory

JANUARY 14TH

May you live all the days of your life.

Jonathan Swift

JANUARY 15TH

Our life is what our thoughts make it.

Marcus Aurelius

JANUARY 16TH

One of the greatest gifts God has given you

is the ability to enjoy pleasure…

He wants you to enjoy life, not just endure it.

Rick Warren

JANUARY 17TH

You can't do anything about the length of your life,

but you can do something about its width and depth.

H.L. Mencken

JANUARY 18TH

Life is like riding a bike.

You don't fall off unless you stop pedaling.

Anonymous

JANUARY 19TH

Accept no one's definition of your life,

but define yourself.

Harvey Fierstein

JANUARY 20TH

All the animals except for man

know that the principle business of life is to enjoy it.

Samuel Butler

JANUARY 21ST

The enjoyment of the journey comes by learning

to love myself despite my imperfection,

limitations and vulnerabilities.

Marge Schneider

JANUARY 22ND

Life is short. Eat dessert first.

Anonymous

JANUARY 23RD

People say that what we're all seeking

is a meaning for life…

I think what we're seeking

is an experience of being alive,

so that our experiences on the purely physical plane will

have resonance within our innermost being and reality,

so that we can actually feel the rapture of being alive.

Joseph Campbell

JANUARY 24TH

Life is too deep for words,

so don't try to describe it, just live it.

C.S. Lewis

JANUARY 25TH

We always have enough to be happy if

we are enjoying what we do have –

and not worrying about what we don't have.

Ken Keyes

JANUARY 26TH

It's not the load that breaks you down,

it's how you carry it.

Lena Horne

JANUARY 27TH

You're only here for a short visit.

Don't hurry. Don't worry.

And be sure to smell the flowers along the way.

Walter Hagen

JANUARY 28TH

The art of life isn't controlling what happens,

which is impossible;

it's using what happens.

Gloria Steinem

JANUARY 29TH

Each person has his or her own purpose and

distinct path, unique and separate from anyone else's.

As you travel your life path, you will be presented with

numerous lessons that you will need to learn in order to

fulfill that purpose. The lessons you are presented with

are specific to you; learning these lessons is the key

to discovering and fulfilling the meaning

and relevance of your life.

Cherie Carter Scott

JANUARY 30TH

The principle of life is that life responds by

corresponding; your life becomes the thing

you have decided it shall be.

Raymond Charles Barker

JANUARY 31ST

Some folks go through life pleased

that the glass is half full.

Others spend a lifetime lamenting

that it's half-empty.

The truth is, there is a glass

with a certain volume of liquid in it.

From there, it's up to you!

James S. Vuocolo

FEBRUARY

FEBRUARY 1ST

The secret of life is not to do what you like

but to like what you do.

Anonymous

FEBRUARY 2ND

It is good to have an end to journey toward;

but it is the journey that matters, in the end.

Ursula K. Le Guin

FEBRUARY 3RD

Learn to wish that everything shall come to pass

exactly as it does.

Epictetus

FEBRUARY 4TH

How we spend our days is, of course,

how we spend our lives.

Annie Dillard

FEBRUARY 5th

What we are today

comes from our thoughts of yesterday,

and our present thoughts build our life of tomorrow.

Our life is the creation of our mind.

Buddha

FEBRUARY 6TH

Be not afraid of life. Believe that life is worth living,

and your belief will help create that fact.

William James

FEBRUARY 7TH

Let us so live that when we come to die

even the undertaker will be sorry.

Mark Twain

FEBRUARY 8TH

Life is about not knowing, having to change,

taking the moment and making the best of it,

without knowing what's going to happen next.

Delicious ambiguity!

Gilda Radner

FEBRUARY 9TH

Develop an interest in life as you see it;

the people, things, literature, music –

the world is so rich, simply throbbing

with rich treasures, beautiful souls and

interesting people. Forget yourself.

Henry Miller

FEBRUARY 10TH

The art of living is always to make

a good thing out of a bad thing.

E.F. Schumacher

FEBRUARY 11TH

Life is a festival only to the wise.

Ralph Waldo Emerson

FEBRUARY 12TH

The longer I live, the more beautiful life becomes.

Frank Lloyd Wright

FEBRUARY 13TH

It is not the events in our lives that do us in,

but the choices we make about how we come to them,

that brings us joy on the journey.

Carl Hammerschlag

FEBRUARY 14TH

Life is a dance. Squeeze the juice out of each moment

and we find our authentic self.

There is no greater benediction.

Charles Swindoll

FEBRUARY 15TH

Whatever is at the center of our life will be the source

of our security, guidance, wisdom, and power.

Stephen Covey

FEBRUARY 16TH

If one thinks that one is happy,

that is enough to be happy.

Madame De La Fayette

FEBRUARY 17TH

Dancing is no mere translation or abstraction from life;

it is life itself.

Havelock Ellis

FEBRUARY 18TH

First of all, life is a journey…

every experience is here to teach you more fully

how to be who you really are.

Oprah Winfrey

FEBRUARY 19TH

Life is to be enjoyed, not just endured.

Gordon B. Hinckley

FEBRUARY 20TH

No man is a failure who is enjoying life.

William Feather

FEBRUARY 21ST

The important thing in life is not to have a good hand

but to play it well.

Louis N. Fortin

FEBRUARY 22ND

Life is a succession of experiences sprinkled

with emotions, people, places, adventures,

triumphs, wonders, disappointments, puzzlements,

injustices, loves, and, if you pay attention,

lessons that make the journey that much more

savory and easily navigable along the way.

Erika Lenkert

FEBRUARY 23RD

The most wasted of all days is that during which

one has not laughed.

Nicolas De Chamfort

FEBRUARY 24TH

We will often find compensation if we think more

of what life has given us and less

about what life has taken away.

William Barclay

FEBRUARY 25TH

Life is like a mirror.

You frown at it, it glares back at you;

you smile at life and it returns the smile.

Ralph Ranson

FEBRUARY 26TH

If we really want to live we must have the courage to

recognize that life is ultimately very short

and that everything we do counts.

When it is the evening of our life we will hopefully

have a chance to look back and say:

"It was worthwhile because I have really lived."

Elisabeth Kübler-Ross

FEBRUARY 27TH

And we should consider every day lost on which

we have not danced at least once.

Friedrich Nietzsche

FEBRUARY 28TH

The art of living is the highest calling of all.

If we start seeing our life as a work of art-in-progress,

we will find that our attitude toward

our life will change.

Alexandra Stoddard

MARCH

MARCH 1ST

Too many people are thinking of

security instead of opportunity.

They seem to be more afraid of life than death.

James F. Bymes

MARCH 2ND

There are two ways to approach life –

as a victim or as a gallant fighter.

Merle Shain

MARCH 3RD

Life should be lived so vividly and so intensely that

thoughts of another life, or of a longer life,

are not necessary.

Marjory Stoneman

MARCH 4TH

The person who has lived the most

is not the one with the most years,

but the one with the richest experiences.

Jean-Jacques Rousseau

MARCH 5TH

I find that when we really love and accept and approve

of ourselves exactly as we are,

then everything in life works.

Louise Hay

MARCH 6TH

To enjoy life more fully

you must keep reminding yourself

that life is too short to waste on unhappiness.

Harold Brecher

MARCH 7TH

The art of life is to know how to enjoy a little

and to endure much.

William Hazlitt

MARCH 8TH

We are all here for a spell;

get all the good laughs you can.

Will Rogers

MARCH 9TH

It's better to light a candle

than to curse the darkness.

Chinese Proverb

MARCH 10TH

Life is like a game of cards.

The hand that is dealt you represents determinism;

the way you play it is free will.

Jawaharlal Nehru

MARCH 11TH

We live in deeds, not years; in thoughts, not breaths;

In feelings, not figures on a dial.

Aristotle

MARCH 12TH

We should count time by heart-throbs.

He most lives who thinks most,

feels the noblest,

acts the best.

Philip James Bailey

MARCH 13TH

Write it on your heart that every day

is the best day of the year.

Ralph Waldo Emerson

MARCH 14TH

Only when we are no longer afraid do we begin to live.

Dorothy Thompson

MARCH 15TH

However mean your life is, meet it and live.

Do not shun it and call it hard names.

It is not so bad as you are.

It looks poorest when you are richest.

The faultfinder will find faults even in paradise.

Love your life, poor as it is.

You may perchance have pleasant, thrilling,

glorious hours, even in a poorhouse.

Henry David Thoreau

MARCH 16TH

The greatest act of revolution in contemporary life,

is to come to every day with joy.

Carl Hammerschlag

MARCH 17TH

What we call the secret of happiness is no more a secret

than our willingness to choose life.

Leo Buscaglia

MARCH 18TH

Life isn't a matter of milestones, but of moments.

Rose Kennedy

MARCH 19TH

The absolute value of love makes life worthwhile,

and so Man's strange and difficult situation acceptable.

Love cannot save life from death;

but it can fulfill life's purpose.

Arnold Toynbee

MARCH 20TH

Is not life a hundred times too short

for us to bore ourselves?

Friedrich Nietzsche

MARCH 21ST

I am beginning to learn that it is the sweet,

simple things of life which are the real ones after all.

Laura Ingalls Wilder

MARCH 22ND

Man is born to live,

not to prepare for life.

Boris Pasternak

MARCH 23RD

It is not that there is no evil, accidents, deformity,

pettiness, hatred. It's that there is a broader view.

Evil exists in the part. Perfection exists in the while.

Discord is seeing near-sightedly.

And I can choose this broader view –

not that I always should – but I always can.

Hugh Prather

MARCH 24TH

Live all you can: it's a mistake not to.

It doesn't much matter what you do in particular,

so long as you have had your life.

If you haven't had that, what have you had?

Henry James

MARCH 25TH

Life is too tragic for sadness. Let us rejoice.

Edward Abbey

MARCH 26TH

We are born not to survive.

Only to live.

W.S. Merwin

MARCH 27TH

Life is no brief candle to me. It is a sort of splendid torch

which I have got a hold of for the moment,

and I want to make it burn as brightly as possible

before handing it onto future generations.

George Bernard Shaw

MARCH 28TH

Life is like a ten-speed bike.

Most of us have gears we never use.

Charles Schulz

MARCH 29TH

Life is a great big canvas;

throw all the paint on it you can.

Danny Kaye

MARCH 30TH

There is no sure for birth or death,

save to enjoy the interval.

George Santayana

MARCH 31ST

Always laugh when you can.

It is cheap medicine.

Lord Byron

APRIL

APRIL 1ST

Dost thou love life? Then do not squander time,

for that's the stuff life is made of.

Benjamin Franklin

APRIL 2ND

Life is like a blanket too short.

You pull it up and your toes rebel,

you yank it down and shivers

meander about your shoulder;

but cheerful folks manage to draw their knees up

and pass a very comfortable night.

Marion Howard

APRIL 3RD

Life is not the way it's supposed to be. It's the way it is.

The way you cope with it is what makes the difference.

Virginia Satir

APRIL 4TH

Even if the patterns of my life

do not conform to my preconceived vision of how

I wished or expected things to be,

every moment is a learning opportunity.

Every moment is sacred.

Every moment offers me a unique challenge.

And, no matter how much I may protest,

every moment is perfect for me at that time.

Jeffrey Mishlove

APRIL 5TH

Everyone dies, but not everyone fully lives.

Anonymous

APRIL 6TH

If you're too busy to enjoy life, you're too busy.

Jeff Davidson

APRIL 7TH

I think of life itself, now, as a wonderful play

that I've written for myself…

And so my purpose is to have

the most fun playing my part.

Shirley MacLaine

APRIL 8TH

I decided long ago never to look at the

right hand of the menu or the price tag of clothes –

otherwise I would starve, naked.

Helen Hayes

APRIL 9TH

That man is a success who has

lived well, laughed often and loved much.

Robert Louis Stevenson

APRIL 10TH

Do not take life too seriously.

You will never get out of it alive.

Elbert Hubbard

APRIL 11TH

Life is 10 percent what happens to me

and 90 percent how I react to it.

Lou Holtz

APRIL 12TH

All I can say about life is, Oh God, enjoy it!

Bob Newhart

APRIL 13TH

Life is a jest; and all things show it.

I thought so once;

but now I know it.

John Gay

APRIL 14TH

True life lies in laughter, love and work.

Elbert Hubbard

APRIL 15TH

Be glad of life because it gives you the chance to love,

and to work, and to play and to look up at the stars.

Henry Van Dyke

APRIL 16TH

One should sympathize with

the joy, the beauty, the color of life –

the less said about life's sores the better.

Oscar Wilde

APRIL 17TH

Take time to laugh, cry and be silent.

Pratigo Dove

APRIL 18TH

So much sadness exists in the world that we are all

under obligation to contribute as much joy

as lies within our powers.

John Sutherland Bonnell

APRIL 19TH

It's a funny thing about life;

if you refuse to accept anything but the best,

you may often get it.

W. Somerset Maugham

APRIL 20TH

The happiness of your life depends upon

the quality of your thoughts.

Marcus Antonius

APRIL 21ST

The greatest discovery of any generation is that

human beings can altar their lives

by altering their attitudes.

Albert Schweitzer

APRIL 22ND

The secret of life is play.

Play and humor are what refines and enhances our joy.

Susan Scott

APRIL 23RD

The grand essentials to happiness in this life are

something to do, something to love

and something to hope for.

Joseph Addison

APRIL 24TH

We act as though comfort and luxury were the chief

requirements of life, when all that we need to make us

really happy is something to be enthusiastic about.

Charles Kingsley

APRIL 25TH

Life is a paradise for those who

love many things with a passion.

Leo Buscaglia

APRIL 26TH

Don't worry, be happy

Meyer Baba

APRIL 27TH

The secret of man's being

is not only to live,

but to have something to live for.

Fyodor Dostoyevsky

APRIL 28TH

The highest form of bliss

is living with a certain degree of folly.

Erasmus

APRIL 29TH

I have very strong feelings about how you lead your life.

You always look ahead,

you never look back.

Ann Richards

APRIL 30TH

The best way to prepare for life is to begin to live.

Elbert Hubbard

MAY

MAY 1ST

Life is the greatest of all bargains; you get it for nothing.

Yiddish Saying

MAY 2ND

The purpose of life is a life of purpose.

Robert Byrne

MAY 3RD

We make a living by what we get,

but we make a life by what we give.

Winston Churchill

MAY 4TH

Life's not always fair.

Sometimes you can get a splinter

even sliding down a rainbow.

Cherralea Morgen

MAY 5TH

Life is about authenticity,

recognizing and honoring one's song,

getting in tune with that song

and singing it well.

Marge Schneider

MAY 6TH

There is more to life than having everything!

Maurice Sendak

MAY 7TH

In three words I can sum up

everything I've learned about life.

It goes on.

Robert Frost

MAY 8TH

Enjoy the little things in life,

for one day you may look back and realize

they were the big things.

Anonymous

MAY 9TH

Life is about dancing together or dancing apart

but just keep dancing.

Nicole Schapiro

MAY 10TH

Live life so completely

that when death comes to you like a thief in the night,

there will be nothing left for him to steal.

Anonymous

MAY 11TH

One of the secrets of a happy life

is continuous small treats.

Iris Murdoch

MAY 12TH

Love the moment

and the energy of that moment will spread

beyond all boundaries into blissful, peaceful happiness.

Corita Kent

MAY 13TH

My advice to you is not to inquire why or whither,

but just enjoy your ice cream while it's on your plate.

Thornton Wilder

MAY 14TH

There are two things to aim at in life:

first, to get what you want;

and, after that, to enjoy it.

Only the wisest of mankind achieve the second.

Logan Pearsall Smith

MAY 15TH

I finally figured out the only reason to be alive

is to enjoy it.

Rita Mae Brown

MAY 16TH

I have found life an enjoyable, enchanting,

active, and sometime terrifying experience,

and I've enjoyed it completely.

A lament in one ear, maybe,

but always a song in the other.

Sean O'Casey

MAY 17TH

Every day we should hear at least one little song,

read one good poem, see one exquisite picture,

and, if possible, speak a few sensible words.

Johann Wolfgang von Goethe

MAY 18TH

Life engenders life.

Energy creates energy.

It is by spending oneself that one becomes rich.

Sarah Bernhardt

MAY 19TH

Live as if you expected to live a hundred years,

but might die tomorrow.

Ann Lee

MAY 20TH

Beginning today, treat everyone you meet as if

they were going to be dead by midnight.

Extend to them all the care, kindness,

and understanding you can muster,

and do it with no thought of any reward.

Your life will never be the same again.

Og Mandino

MAY 21ST

Life is just a blank slate,

what matters most is what you write on it.

Christine Frankland

MAY 22ND

Like fireworks, this universe is a celebration

and you are the spectator contemplating the eternal

Fourth of July of your absolute splendor.

Francis Lucille

MAY 23RD

Most of the shadows of this life

are caused by our standing in our own sunshine.

Ralph Waldo Emerson

MAY 24TH

The world is a mirror: what looks in looks out.

It gives back only what you lend it.

Ludwig Boeme

MAY 25TH

The purpose of life, after all, is to live it,

to taste experience to the utmost,

to reach out eagerly and without fear

for newer and richer experiences.

Eleanor Roosevelt

MAY 26TH

The follies which a person regrets most in his life

are those he didn't commit

when he had the opportunity.

Helen Rowland

MAY 27TH

Twenty years from now you will be

more disappointed by the things

that you didn't do than by the ones you did do.

So throw off the bowlines.

Sail away from the safe harbor.

Catch the trade winds in your sails.

Explore. Dream. Discover.

Mark Twain

MAY 28TH

Live in such a way that you would not be ashamed

to sell your parrot to the town gossip.

Will Rogers

MAY 29TH

There are only two ways to live your life.

One is as though nothing is a miracle.

The other is as though everything is a miracle.

Albert Einstein

MAY 30TH

The art of being happy lies in the power

of extracting happiness from common things.

Henry Ward Beecher

MAY 31ST

Anyone can be happy when times are good;

the richer experience is to be happy when times are not.

Susan Harris

JUNE

JUNE 1ST

All the wonderful things in life are so simple

that one is not aware of their wonder

until they are beyond touch.

Frances Gunther

JUNE 2ND

Life is the art of drawing without an eraser.

John W. Gardner

JUNE 3RD

If we could see the miracle of a single flower clearly

our whole life would change.

Buddha

JUNE 4TH

We win half the battle when we make up our minds
to take the world as we find it, including the thorns.

Orison S. Marden

JUNE 5TH

Ah, the smell of flowers. I've just put flowers in a vase.
The meaning of life is the flowers in the vase.

Helen Caldicott

JUNE 6TH

Lightness of touch and living in the moment are
intertwined. One cannot dance well
unless one is completely in time with the music,
not leaning back to the last step
or pressing forward to the next one,
but poised directly on the present step as it comes.

Anne Morrow Lindbergh

JUNE 7TH

Life is a child playing around your feet,

a tool you hold firmly in your grip,

a bench you sit down upon in the evening,

in your garden.

Jean Anouilh

JUNE 8TH

You don't get to choose how you're going to die.

Or when.

You can only decide how you're going to live.

Now.

Joan Baez

JUNE 9TH

The best things in life are nearest:

Breath in your nostrils, light in your eyes,

flowers at your feet, duties at your hand,

the path of right just before you.

Then do not grasp at the stars, but do life's plain,

common work as it comes,

certain that daily duties and daily bread

are the sweetest things in life.

Robert Louis Stevenson

JUNE 10TH

Each day of your life, as soon as you open your eyes in

the morning, you can square away

for a happy and successful day.

George Matthew Adams

JUNE 11TH

Normal day, let me be aware of the treasure you are.

Mary Jean Irion

JUNE 12TH

To be alive, to be able to see, to walk…

it's all a miracle.

Arthur Rubinstein

JUNE 13TH

The secret of life is to have a task, something you devote

your entire life to, something you bring everything to,

every minute of the day for the rest of your life.

And the most important thing is,

it must be something you cannot possibly do.

Henry Moore

JUNE 14TH

We are continually faced with great opportunities

which are brilliantly disguised as unsolvable problems.

Margaret Mead

JUNE 15TH

Greet each day with your eyes open to beauty,

your mind open to change,

and your heart open to love.

Paula Finn

JUNE 16TH

The past is gone, the future is not yet here,

and if we do not go back to ourselves in the present

moment, we cannot be in touch with life.

Thich Nhat Hann

JUNE 17TH

I don't think of all the misery

but of the beauty that still remains.

Anne Frank

JUNE 18TH

So never let a cloudy day ruin your sunshine,

for even if you can't see it, the sunshine is still there,

inside of you ready to shine when you let it.

Amy Pitzele

JUNE 19TH

He who has the why to live

can bear with almost any how.

Friedrich Nietzsche

JUNE 20TH

Getting born is like being given a ticket to

the theatrical event called life.

Now, all that ticket will get you is through the door.

It doesn't get you a good time

and it doesn't get you a bad time.

You go in and sit down and you either

love the show or you don't. If you do, terrific.

And if you don't – that's show business.

Stewart Emery

JUNE 21ST

Life is the sum of all your choices.

Albert Camus

JUNE 22ND

Don't wait around for other people to be happy for you.

Any happiness you get you've got to make yourself.

Alice Walker

JUNE 23RD

My Mama always said life was like a box of chocolates.

You never know what you're gonna get.

Tom Hanks in Forest Gump

JUNE 24TH

The last of human freedoms –

to choose one's attitude

in any given set of circumstances,

to choose one's way.

Viktor Frankl

JUNE 25TH

If you can spend a perfectly useless afternoon

in a perfectly useless manner,

you have learned how to live.

Lin Yutang

JUNE 26TH

Live each day as if your life had just begun.

Johann Wolfgang von Goethe

JUNE 27TH

Life is a grindstone.

Whether it grinds us down or polishes us up

depends on us.

L. Thomas Holdcroft

JUNE 28TH

We live in a wonderful world that is full

of beauty, charm and adventure.

There is no end to the adventures that we can have

if only we seek them with our eyes open.

Jawaharlal Nehru

JUNE 29TH

Every day is a good day.

Yun-Men

JUNE 30TH

Yesterday is ashes tomorrow wood.

Only today does the fire burn brightly.

Eskimo Saying

JULY

JULY 1ST

Life is a succession of moments.

To live each one is to succeed.

Coretta Scott King

JULY 2ND

Stop worrying about the potholes in the road

and celebrate the journey!

Barbara Hoffman

JULY 3RD

The only way to live is to accept each minute as an

unrepeatable miracle, which is exactly what it is:

a miracle and unrepeatable.

Storm Jameson

JULY 4TH

Life is a roller coaster. Try to eat a light lunch.

David A. Schmaltz

JULY 5TH

Look, I really don't want to wax philosophical,

but I will say that if you're alive,

you got to flap your arms and legs,

you got to jump around a lot, you got to make a lot

of noise, because life is the very opposite of death.

And therefore, as I see it, if you're quiet,

you're not living.

You've got to be noisy or at least your thoughts

should be noisy and colorful and lively.

Mel Brooks

JULY 6TH

Morning is when I am awake and there is dawn in me.

Henry David Thoreau

JULY 7TH

The ideals which have lighted my way,

and time after time have given me

new courage to face life cheerfully,

have been Kindness, Beauty, and Truth...

Albert Einstein

JULY 8TH

Today, this hour, this minute is the day, the hour, the

minute for each of us to sense the fact that life is good,

with all it's trials and troubles, and perhaps

more interesting because of them.

Robert Updegraff

JULY 9TH

Life is not a problem to be solved but a gift to be opened.

Wayne Muller

JULY 10TH

Wherever you go, no matter what the weather,

always bring your own sunshine.

Anthony J. D'Angelo

JULY 11TH

Nothing should be more highly prized

than the value of each day.

Johann Wolfgang von Goethe

JULY 12TH

One of the most tragic things I know about human

nature is that all of us tend to put off living.

We are all dreaming of some magical rose garden over

the horizon – instead of enjoying the roses

blooming outside our windows today.

Dale Carnegie

JULY 13TH

Be happy in the moment – that's enough.

Each moment is all we need – not more.

Mother Teresa

JULY 14TH

If you are not playful you are not alive.

David Hockney

JULY 15TH

I don't want to get to the end of my life and find

that I have just lived the length of it.

I want to have lived the width of it as well.

Diane Ackerman

JULY 16TH

Strong lives are motivated by dynamic purposes.

Kenneth Hildebrand

JULY 17TH

Why not go out on a limb?

Isn't that where the fruit is?

Frank Scully

JULY 18TH

Jump into the middle of things,

get your hands dirty,

fall flat on your face,

and then reach for the stars.

Joan L. Curcio

JULY 19TH

Let the day be lost to us

on which we did not dance once!

Friedrich Nietzsche

JULY 20TH

Live as you will have wished to have lived

when you are dying.

Christian Furchtegott Gellert

JULY 21ST

Time is the coin of your life.

It is the only coin you have,

and only you can determine how it will be spent.

Be careful lest you let other people spend it for you.

Carl Sandburg

JULY 22ND

When making your choice in life, do not neglect to live.

Samuel Johnson

JULY 23RD

Do not look back on happiness or dream of it

in the future. You are only sure of today;

do not let yourself be cheated out of it.

Henry Ward Beecher

JULY 24TH

Life is a mixed blessing,

which we vainly try to unmix.

Mignon McLaughlin

91

JULY 25TH

Grab a chance and you won't be sorry

for a might-have-been.

Arthur Mitchell Ransome

JULY 26TH

The whole world is an art gallery when you're mindful.

There are beautiful things everywhere –

and they're free.

Charles Tart

JULY 27TH

The world is its own magic.

Shunryu Suzuki

JULY 28TH

Sooner or later we all discover that

the important moments in life

are not the advertised ones, not the birthdays,

the graduations, the weddings,

not the great goals achieved.

The real milestones are less prepossessing.

They come to the

door of memory unannounced,

stray dogs that amble in,

sniff around a bit and simply never leave.

Our lives are measured by these.

Susan B. Anthony

JULY 29TH

If we are ever to enjoy life, now is the time,

not tomorrow or next year…

Today should always be our most wonderful day.

Thomas Dreier

JULY 30TH

Never again clutter your days or nights with so many

menial and unimportant things that you have no time

to accept a real challenge when it comes along.

This applies to play as well as work.

A day merely survived is no cause for celebration.

You are not here to fritter away your precious hours

when you have the ability to accomplish so much

by making a slight change in your routine.

No more busy work. No more hiding from success.

Leave time, leave space, to grow.

Now. Now! Not tomorrow!

Og Mandino

JULY 31ST

It is only possible to live happily ever after

on a day-to-day basis.

Margaret Bonanno

AUGUST

AUGUST 1ST

The past is behind, learn from it;

The future is ahead, prepare for it;

The present is here, live in it.

Thomas Monson

AUGUST 2ND

Take the reins of your life in your hands every day.

Get up and put a smile on your face,

and feel grateful for this gift that is your life.

Susan L. Taylor

AUGUST 3RD

Each day comes bearing it's own gifts.

Untie the ribbons.

Ruth Ann Schabacker

August 4th

I live a day at a time.

Each day I look for a kernel of excitement.

In the morning, I say:

"What is my exciting thing for today?"

Then, I do the day.

Don't ask me about tomorrow.

Barbara Jordan

August 5th

Learn to enjoy every minute of your life. Be happy now.

Don't wait for something outside of yourself

to make you happy in the future.

Think how really precious is the time you have to spend,

whether it's at work or with your family.

Every minute should be enjoyed and savored.

Earl Nightingale

AUGUST 6TH

Accept the challenges, so that you may feel the

exhilaration of victory.

General George S. Patton

AUGUST 7TH

Look at each day as a chance to invest life into life.

A chance to share your experience

and deposit it into someone else's conscience.

Each day is a chance to work miracles

in the lives of others.

Jim Rohn

AUGUST 8TH

Dare to live the life you have dreamed for yourself.

Go forward and make your dreams come true.

Ralph Waldo Emerson

AUGUST 9TH

Be not afraid of life. Believe that life is worth living

and your belief will help create the fact.

William James

AUGUST 10TH

Life is lived in the present.

Yesterday is gone.

Tomorrow is yet to be.

Today is the miracle.

Anonymous

AUGUST 11TH

Nothing is worth more than this day.

Johann Wolfgang von Goethe

AUGUST 12TH

Seize every day as an adventure

and your spirit will soar when you discover

the wonderful surprises life has to offer.

Anonymous

AUGUST 13TH

Life can only be understood backwards;

but it must be lived forwards.

Soren Kierkegaard

AUGUST 14TH

Be not forgetful to cherish the gifts each moment brings.

Anonymous

AUGUST 15TH

Live in the present moment and find your

interest and happiness in the things of today.

Emmett Fox

AUGUST 16TH

He who lives in harmony with himself

lives in harmony with the world.

Marcus Aurelius

AUGUST 17TH

It's all a miracle.

I have adopted the technique of living life

from miracle to miracle.

Arthur Rubinstein

AUGUST 18TH

Dwell as near as possible to the channel

in which your life flows.

Henry David Thoreau

AUGUST 19TH

The only way to have a life is to commit to it like crazy.

Angelina Jolie

AUGUST 20TH

He who has nothing to die for

has nothing to live for.

Moroccan Proverb

AUGUST 21ST

When you were born,

you cried and the world rejoiced.

Live your life so that when you die,

the world cries and you rejoice.

Cherokee Expression

AUGUST 22ND

Life is a promise; fulfill it.

Mother Teresa

AUGUST 23RD

Purpose serves as a principle

around which to organize our lives.

Anonymous

AUGUST 24TH

The greatest risk is the risk of riskless living.

Stephen Covey

AUGUST 25TH

Find a purpose in life so big

that it will challenge every capacity to be at your best.

David O. McKay

August 26th

There is no such thing in anyone's life

as an unimportant day.

Alexander Woollcott

August 27th

Life is a great and wondrous mystery

and the only thing we know that we have for sure

is what is right here right now. Don't miss it.

Leo Buscaglia

August 28th

In the book of life, the answers aren't in the back.

Charles Schulz

AUGUST 29TH

The meaning of life?

It is life itself.

Marek Halter

AUGUST 30TH

Life is a celebration of being here on earth.

Margie Klein

AUGUST 31ST

Just living is not enough.

One must have sunshine, freedom,

and a little flower.

Hans Christian Anderson

SEPTEMBER

SEPTEMBER 1ST

When I stand before God at the end of my life,

I would hope that I would not have

a single bit of talent left, and could say,

"I used everything you gave me."

Erma Bombeck

SEPTEMBER 2ND

The miracle is not to fly in the air,

or to walk on the water,

but to walk on the earth.

Chinese Proverb

SEPTEMBER 3RD

Life is simple, it's just not easy.

Anonymous

SEPTEMBER 4TH

A life without cause is a life without effect.

Barbarella

SEPTEMBER 5TH

Life is like a beautiful melody,

only the lyrics are messed up.

Anonymous

SEPTEMBER 6TH

Here is the test to find

whether your mission on earth is finished.

If you're alive, it isn't.

Richard Bach

SEPTEMBER 7TH

Life leaps like a geyser

for those willing to drill through the rock of inertia.

Alexis Carrel

SEPTEMBER 8TH

As we struggle to make sense of things,

life looks on in repose.

Anonymous

SEPTEMBER 9TH

I have a simple philosophy:

Fill what's empty. Empty what's full.

Scratch where it itches.

Alice Roosevelt Longworth

SEPTEMBER 10TH

Life is like a coin.

You can spend it any way you wish,

but you only spend it once.

Lillian Dickson

SEPTEMBER 11TH

God pours life into death and death into life

without a drop being spilled.

Anonymous

SEPTEMBER 12TH

Life is what we make it,

always has been, always will be.

Grandma Moses

SEPTEMBER 13TH

Who will tell whether one happy moment of love

or the joy of breathing or walking on a bright morning

and smelling the fresh air, is not worth

all the suffering and effort which life implies.

Erich Fromm

SEPTEMBER 14TH

Life is a ticket to the greatest show on earth.

Martin H. Fischer

SEPTEMBER 15TH

To live remains an art which everyone must learn,

and which no one can teach.

Havelock Ellis

SEPTEMBER 16TH

Living involves tearing up one rough draft after another.

Anonymous

SEPTEMBER 17TH

My grandfather always said that living is like

licking honey off a thorn.

Louis Adamic

SEPTEMBER 18TH

No man lives without jostling and being jostled;

in all ways he has to elbow himself through the world,

giving and receiving offence.

Thomas Carlyle

SEPTEMBER 19TH

Don't think of retiring from the world

until the world will be sorry that you retire.

I hate a fellow whom pride or cowardice or

laziness drive into a corner, and who does nothing

when he is there but sit and growl.

Let him come out as I do, and bark.

Samuel Johnson

SEPTEMBER 20TH

Life loves to be taken by the lapel and told:

"I am with you kid. Let's go."

Maya Angelou

SEPTEMBER 21ST

Don't go around saying the world owes you a living.

The world owes you nothing. It was here first.

Mark Twain

SEPTEMBER 22ND

Life has meaning only if one barters it day by day

for something other than itself.

Antoine de Saint-Exupery

SEPTEMBER 23RD

You will never be happy if you

continue to search for what happiness consists of.

You will never live if you

are looking for the meaning of life.

Albert Camus

SEPTEMBER 24TH

There is no wealth but life.

John Ruskin

SEPTEMBER 25TH

The price of anything

is the amount of life you exchange for it.

Henry David Thoreau

SEPTEMBER 26TH

What good are vitamins?

Eat four lobsters, eat a pound of caviar – live!

Arthur Rubinstein

SEPTEMBER 27TH

Life is not a final. It's daily pop quizzes.

Anonymous

SEPTEMBER 28TH

Eating, loving, singing and digesting are, in truth,

the four acts of the comic opera known as life,

and they pass like bubbles of a bottle of champagne.

Whoever lets them break without having enjoyed them

is a complete fool.

Gioacchino Rossini

SEPTEMBER 29TH

Any idiot can face a crisis –

it's day to day living that wears you out.

Anton Chekhov

SEPTEMBER 30TH

Life is so largely controlled by chance that its conduct

can be but a perpetual improvisation.

W. Somerset Maugham

OCTOBER

OCTOBER 1ST

In life we all have an unspeakable secret, an irreversible regret, an unreachable dream and an unforgettable love.

Diego Marchi

OCTOBER 2ND

The philosophy of mine earth can be summed up as this:

Sunshine creates happiness, and I create myself.

Nights are long, and life is predominantly good.

Wind is refreshing.

Tea is wisdom.

Do the best you can, and be good to yourself

so that you can above all

be good to others.

Jessi Lane Adams

OCTOBER 3RD

Human life is purely a matter of

deciding what's important to you.

Anonymous

OCTOBER 4TH

For if there is a sin against life, it consists perhaps

not so much in despairing of life

as in hoping for another life and in eluding

the implacable grandeur of this life.

Albert Camus

OCTOBER 5TH

Life is a compromise of what your ego wants to do,

what experience tells you to do,

and what your nerves let you do.

Bruce Crampton

OCTOBER 6TH

To succeed in life, you need three things:

a wishbone,

a backbone,

and a funnybone.

Reba McEntire

OCTOBER 7TH

The tragedy of life is not so much what men suffer,

but rather what they miss.

Thomas Carlyle

OCTOBER 8TH

All the art of living lies in a fine mingling

of letting go and holding on.

Havelock Ellis

OCTOBER 9TH

We're all accidental soldiers in the army of life.

Ymber Delecto

OCTOBER 10TH

To look back all the time is boring.

Excitement lies in tomorrow.

Natalia Makrova

OCTOBER 11TH

God asks no man whether he will accept life.

That is not the choice. You must take it.

The only question is how.

Henry Ward Beecher

OCTOBER 12TH

Life is a train of moods like a string of beads;

and as we pass through them

they prove to be many colored lenses,

which paint the world their own hue,

and each shows us only what lies in its own face.

Ralph Waldo Emerson

OCTOBER 13TH

Suppose the world were only one of God's jokes,

would you work any the less to make it

a good joke instead of a bad one?

George Bernard Shaw

OCTOBER 14TH

Life is just a collection of memories...

but memories, my friends, are like starlight

because memories go on forever.

C.W. McCall

OCTOBER 15TH

Live your life each day, as you would climb a mountain.

An occasional glance towards the summit keeps the goal

in mind, but many beautiful scenes are to be observed

from each new vantage point.

Harold B. Melchant

OCTOBER 16TH

It may be life is only worthwhile at moments.

Perhaps that is all we ought to expect.

Sherwood Anderson

OCTOBER 17TH

Life is not measured by the number of breaths we take,

but by the moments that take our breath away.

Anonymous

OCTOBER 18TH

Serenity of spirit and turbulence of action

should make up the sum of a man's life.

Vita Sackville-West

OCTOBER 19TH

You live and learn.

At any rate, you live.

Douglas Adams

OCTOBER 20TH

Life is made up of constant calls to action,

and we seldom have time for more than

hastily contrived answers.

Learned Hand

OCTOBER 21ST

The true harvest of my daily life is

somewhat as intangible and indescribable

as the tints of morning or evening.

It is a little star dust caught,

a segment of the rainbow which I have clutched.

Henry David Thoreau

OCTOBER 22ND

Life is an enjoyable game to be played –

not a horrible problem to be solved.

Ken Keyes

OCTOBER 23RD

The aim of life is to live,

and to live means to be aware,

joyously, drunkenly, serenely, divinely aware.

Henry Miller

OCTOBER 24TH

Life isn't all about what you don't have, but yet,

what you do with what you have been given.

Robert M. Hensel

OCTOBER 25TH

Few of us write great novels;

all of us live them.

Mignon McLaughlin

OCTOBER 26TH

Life just is. You have to flow with it.

Give yourself to the moment. Let it happen.

Jerry Brown

OCTOBER 27TH

Sometimes questions are more important than answers.

Nancy Willard

OCTOBER 28TH

It is while you are patiently toiling

at the little tasks of life

that the meaning and shape of the great whole of life

dawn on you.

Phillips Brooks

OCTOBER 29TH

If a man in the morning hear the right way,

he may die in the evening without regret.

Confucius

OCTOBER 30TH

In small proportions we just beauties see;

And in short measures life may perfect be.

Ben Jonson

OCTOBER 31ST

Life always bursts the boundaries of formulas.

Antoine de Saint-Exupéry

NOVEMBER

NOVEMBER 1ST

Life is not having been told

that the man has just waxed the floor.

Ogden Nash

NOVEMBER 2ND

It is completely usual for me

to get up in the morning,

take a look around,

and laugh out loud.

Barbara Kingsolver

NOVEMBER 3RD

Life is a long lesson in humility.

James M. Barrie

NOVEMBER 4TH

In life, as in restaurants, we swallow a lot of indigestible

stuff just because it comes with the dinner.

Mignon McLaughlin

NOVEMBER 5TH

To live is like to love –

all reason is against it, and all healthy instinct for it.

Samuel Butler

NOVEMBER 6TH

Life is easier than you'd think;

all that is necessary is to accept the impossible,

do without the indispensable, and bear the intolerable.

Kathleen Norris

NOVEMBER 7TH

There are people who so arrange their lives

that they feed themselves only on side dishes.

José Ortega y Gasset

NOVEMBER 8TH

The universe is like a safe

to which there is a combination.

But the combination is locked up in the safe.

Peter De Vries

NOVEMBER 9TH

A great part of life consists in contemplating

what we cannot cure.

Robert Louis Stevenson

NOVEMBER 10TH

Chance is always powerful,

let your hook always be cast;

in the pool where you least expect it,

there will be a fish.

Ovid

NOVEMBER 11TH

Living in the past is a dull and lonely business;

looking back strains the neck muscles,

causes you to bump into people not going your way.

Edna Ferber

135

NOVEMBER 12TH

One must never lose time in vanity regretting the past

nor in complaining about the changes

which cause us discomfort,

for change is the very essence of life.

Antole France

NOVEMBER 13TH

Expecting the world to treat you fairly

because you are good

is like expecting the bull not to charge

because you are a vegetarian.

Dennis Wholey

NOVEMBER 14TH

Life is an endless struggle

full of frustrations and challenges,

but eventually you find a hair stylist you like.

Anonymous

NOVEMBER 15TH

I have learned to live each day as it comes,

and not to borrow trouble by dreading tomorrow.

Dorothy Dix

NOVEMBER 16TH

Life, we learn too late, is in the living,

in the tissue of every day and hour.

Stephen Leacock

NOVEMBER 17TH

Unbeing dead isn't being alive.

E.E. Cummings

NOVEMBER 18TH

Think, if you will, of your life as an art gallery

and the events in it as paintings that you have made.

A week ago or a year ago or just yesterday

you began a picture and today

it turns up in the gallery that is your life.

You stop to look at it. Is it beautiful…or is it ugly…?

Whatever it is, see it as a painting

in the gallery of your life,

and consider that the spirit in which you paint today

determines how nice your gallery looks tomorrow.

Brian Browne Walker

NOVEMBER 19TH

I am alive today by the grace of a higher being.

Every day is extra.

John Kerry

NOVEMBER 20TH

Too often life can seem to be

an unpredictable ride between birth and death:

we are born without choosing, and we die at any time.

In between there are many entrances, exits, and detours –

some bring great blessings, others great sorrow.

Yet we always have some degree of choice –

opportunities to fail, or to flourish.

Put yourself in the driver's seat as often as possible,

and stay awake behind the wheel.

Life is a road trip to be experienced to the fullest.

Liam Cunningham

NOVEMBER 21ST

Life is to explore, to discover, to delight

and to be delighted.

Nicole Schapiro

NOVEMBER 22ND

Stop sitting there with your hands folded,

looking on, doing nothing.

Get into action and live this full and glorious life NOW.

You have to do it.

Eileen Caddy

NOVEMBER 23RD

Unrest of spirit is a mark of life

one problem after another presents itself

in the solving of them

we can find our greatest pleasure.

Karl Menninger

NOVEMBER 24TH

Life is made up of desires that seem

big and vital one minute and little and absurd the next.

I guess we get what's best for us in the end.

Alice Caldwell

NOVEMBER 25TH

The difference between life and the movies

is that a script has to make sense, and life doesn't.

Joseph L. Mankiewicz

NOVEMBER 26TH

Be intent upon the perfection of the present day.

William Law

NOVEMBER 27TH

Life is an unfoldment, and the further we travel

the more truth we can comprehend.

To understand the things that are at our door

is the best preparation for understanding

those that lie beyond.

Hypatia

NOVEMBER 28TH

When you stop comparing what is right here and now

with what you wish were,

you can begin to enjoy what is.

Cheri Huber

NOVEMBER 29TH

Life moves pretty fast.

If you don't stop and look around once in a while,

you could miss it.

Matthew Broderick in Ferris Bueller's Day Off

NOVEMBER 30TH

Look. This is your world!

You can't not look..

There is no other world.

This is your world; it is your feast.

You inherited this; you inherited these eyeballs;

you inherited this world of color.

Look at the greatness of the whole thing.

Look! Don't hesitate – look!

Open your eyes.

Don't blink, and look, look – look further.

Chogyam Trungpa

DECEMBER

DECEMBER 1ST

One day at a time – this is enough.

Do not look back and grieve over the past, for it is gone;

and do not be troubled about the future,

for it has not yet come. Live in the present,

and make it so beautiful it will be worth remembering.

Ida Scott Taylor

DECEMBER 2ND

We can discover this meaning in life

in three different ways:

1. by doing a deed;

2. by experiencing a value; and

3. by suffering.

Viktor Frankl

December 3rd

Don't judge each day by the harvest you reap,

but by the seeds you plant.

Robert Louis Stevenson

December 4th

Life is indeed a journey.

We don't have a map unless we draw one up ourselves,

and the road is filled with unknowns.

Sometimes there's smooth sailing,

sometimes there are potholes, detours, washouts,

and never ending sections of major construction.

Sometimes we have to speed up, other times

we need to slow down, stop, wait, and even back up.

But through it all, those of us who truly know how to

live are aware of that, wherever we may be,

it pays to look around and enjoy the scenery.

C. Leslie Charles

DECEMBER 5TH

We're here to feel the joy of life pulsing in us – now.

Joyce Carol Oates

DECEMBER 6TH

I have found that if you love life,

life will love you back.

Arthur Rubinstein

DECEMBER 7TH

A garden is always a series of losses

set against a few triumphs,

like life itself.

May Sarton

DECEMBER 8TH

As we may miss the joy of life by dwelling on the past,

so we miss the possibilities of the present

if we expect life's best days to be in the future.

The good days are now.

Lionel A. Whiston

DECEMBER 9TH

Life is a test, a school where we come to learn and grow

in our spiritual understanding and personal

development, a school designed for each of us to reach

our own unique destiny. Each of us is here to learn, to

grow, to master the challenges that we face,

and to expand our capacity for love and compassion.

Taking life on with courage,

trusting that we are meant to learn

from every experience in life,

is why we are here.

Judy Tatelbaum

DECEMBER 10TH

The whole of life lies in the verb seeing.

Pierre Teilhard De Chardin

DECEMBER 11TH

Life is tough, but I'm tougher.

Andy Rooney

DECEMBER 12TH

The art of living…is neither careless drifting on the one

hand nor fearful clinging to the past on the other.

It consists in being sensitive to each moment,

in regarding it as utterly new and unique,

in having the mind open and wholly receptive.

Alan Watts

DECEMBER

DECEMBER 13TH

If your ship doesn't come in, swim out to it!

John A. Shedd

DECEMBER 14TH

When life fits our expectations,

we think of it as an opportunity.

When it does not, we think

the world failed us, not our expectations.

But that is a mistake,

for life will be whatever it wants to be,

and not necessarily what we want.

Arnold Beisser

DECEMBER 15TH

The art of life

is a constant readjustment to our surroundings.

Kakuzo Okakaura

151

DECEMBER 16TH

Live now, believe me, wait not till tomorrow;

Gather the roses of life today.

Pierre De Ronsard

DECEMBER 17TH

When the days are too short

chances are you are living at your best.

Earl Nightingale

DECEMBER 18TH

Look at life through the windshield,

not the rearview mirror.

Byrd Bagget

DECEMBER 19TH

Life is either a daring adventure or nothing.

Hellen Keller

DECEMBER 20TH

We shall draw from the heart of suffering itself

the means of inspiration and survival.

Winston Churchill

DECEMBER 21ST

Nobody gets to live life backward.

Look ahead –

that's where your future lies.

Ann Landers

DECEMBER 22ND

This – this was what made life: a moment of quiet,

the water falling in the fountain, the girl's voice…

a moment of captured beauty.

He who is truly wise

will never permit such moments to escape.

Louis L'Amour

DECEMBER 23RD

Life is a journey, from birth to death.

If you awake to the possibilities of your journey,

it will lead you from isolation to connection;

from ignorance to knowledge;

from pretense to authenticity;

and from fear to love.

Susan Page

DECEMBER 24TH

I live now and only now, and I will do

what I want to do this moment and not

what I decided was best for me yesterday.

Hugh Prathner

DECEMBER 25TH

We cannot direct the wind

but we can adjust the sails.

Anonymous

DECEMBER 26TH

Life is a series of seconds; a series of events;

a series of opportunities

and a series of life-giving moments.

As we live fully each moment we breathe a fullness

not only into our own life but into the lives

of all we touch and into the very universe itself.

Anne Bryan

DECEMBER 27TH

The highest of wisdom is continual cheerfulness:

such a state, like the region above the moon,

is always clear and serene.

Michel De Montaigne

DECEMBER 28TH

Attitude is a little thing that makes a big difference.

Winston Churchill

DECEMBER 29TH

You gain strength, courage and confidence

by every experience in which

you really stop to look fear in the face.

Eleanor Roosevelt

DECEMBER 30TH

I've got dreams in hidden places

and extra smiles for when I'm blue.

Anonymous

DECEMBER 31ST

There is much in the world to make us afraid.

There is much more in our faith to make us unafraid.

Frederick W. Cropp

www.ingramcontent.com/pod-product-compliance
Lightning Source LLC
Chambersburg PA
CBHW030017290326
41934CB00005B/372